Essay on the Liverpool spa' water, by Thomas Houlston, M.D.

Thomas Houlston

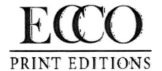

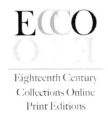

Eighteenth Century
Collections Online
Print Editions

Gale ECCO Print Editions

Relive history with *Eighteenth Century Collections Online*, now available in print for the independent historian and collector. This series includes the most significant English-language and foreign-language works printed in Great Britain during the eighteenth century, and is organized in seven different subject areas including literature and language; medicine, science, and technology; and religion and philosophy. The collection also includes thousands of important works from the Americas.

The eighteenth century has been called "The Age of Enlightenment." It was a period of rapid advance in print culture and publishing, in world exploration, and in the rapid growth of science and technology – all of which had a profound impact on the political and cultural landscape. At the end of the century the American Revolution, French Revolution and Industrial Revolution, perhaps three of the most significant events in modern history, set in motion developments that eventually dominated world political, economic, and social life.

In a groundbreaking effort, Gale initiated a revolution of its own: digitization of epic proportions to preserve these invaluable works in the largest online archive of its kind. Contributions from major world libraries constitute over 175,000 original printed works. Scanned images of the actual pages, rather than transcriptions, recreate the works *as they first appeared.*

Now for the first time, these high-quality digital scans of original works are available via print-on-demand, making them readily accessible to libraries, students, independent scholars, and readers of all ages.

For our initial release we have created seven robust collections to form one the world's most comprehensive catalogs of 18th century works.

Initial Gale ECCO Print Editions collections include:

History and Geography

Rich in titles on English life and social history, this collection spans the world as it was known to eighteenth-century historians and explorers. Titles include a wealth of travel accounts and diaries, histories of nations from throughout the world, and maps and charts of a world that was still being discovered. Students of the War of American Independence will find fascinating accounts from the British side of conflict.

Social Science

Delve into what it was like to live during the eighteenth century by reading the first-hand accounts of everyday people, including city dwellers and farmers, businessmen and bankers, artisans and merchants, artists and their patrons, politicians and their constituents. Original texts make the American, French, and Industrial revolutions vividly contemporary.

Medicine, Science and Technology

Medical theory and practice of the 1700s developed rapidly, as is evidenced by the extensive collection, which includes descriptions of diseases, their conditions, and treatments. Books on science and technology, agriculture, military technology, natural philosophy, even cookbooks, are all contained here.

Literature and Language

Western literary study flows out of eighteenth-century works by Alexander Pope, Daniel Defoe, Henry Fielding, Frances Burney, Denis Diderot, Johann Gottfried Herder, Johann Wolfgang von Goethe, and others. Experience the birth of the modern novel, or compare the development of language using dictionaries and grammar discourses.

Religion and Philosophy

The Age of Enlightenment profoundly enriched religious and philosophical understanding and continues to influence present-day thinking. Works collected here include masterpieces by David Hume, Immanuel Kant, and Jean-Jacques Rousseau, as well as religious sermons and moral debates on the issues of the day, such as the slave trade. The Age of Reason saw conflict between Protestantism and Catholicism transformed into one between faith and logic -- a debate that continues in the twenty-first century.

Law and Reference

This collection reveals the history of English common law and Empire law in a vastly changing world of British expansion. Dominating the legal field is the *Commentaries of the Law of England* by Sir William Blackstone, which first appeared in 1765. Reference works such as almanacs and catalogues continue to educate us by revealing the day-to-day workings of society.

Fine Arts

The eighteenth-century fascination with Greek and Roman antiquity followed the systematic excavation of the ruins at Pompeii and Herculaneum in southern Italy; and after 1750 a neoclassical style dominated all artistic fields. The titles here trace developments in mostly English-language works on painting, sculpture, architecture, music, theater, and other disciplines. Instructional works on musical instruments, catalogs of art objects, comic operas, and more are also included.

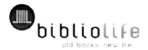

The BiblioLife Network

This project was made possible in part by the BiblioLife Network (BLN), a project aimed at addressing some of the huge challenges facing book preservationists around the world. The BLN includes libraries, library networks, archives, subject matter experts, online communities and library service providers. We believe every book ever published should be available as a high-quality print reproduction; printed on-demand anywhere in the world. This insures the ongoing accessibility of the content and helps generate sustainable revenue for the libraries and organizations that work to preserve these important materials.

The following book is in the "public domain" and represents an authentic reproduction of the text as printed by the original publisher. While we have attempted to accurately maintain the integrity of the original work, there are sometimes problems with the original work or the micro-film from which the books were digitized. This can result in minor errors in reproduction. Possible imperfections include missing and blurred pages, poor pictures, markings and other reproduction issues beyond our control. Because this work is culturally important, we have made it available as part of our commitment to protecting, preserving, and promoting the world's literature.

GUIDE TO FOLD-OUTS MAPS and OVERSIZED IMAGES

The book you are reading was digitized from microfilm captured over the past thirty to forty years. Years after the creation of the original microfilm, the book was converted to digital files and made available in an online database.

In an online database, page images do not need to conform to the size restrictions found in a printed book. When converting these images back into a printed bound book, the page sizes are standardized in ways that maintain the detail of the original. For large images, such as fold-out maps, the original page image is split into two or more pages

Guidelines used to determine how to split the page image follows:

• Some images are split vertically; large images require vertical and horizontal splits.
• For horizontal splits, the content is split left to right.
• For vertical splits, the content is split from top to bottom.
• For both vertical and horizontal splits, the image is processed from top left to bottom right.

ESSAY

ON THE

LIVERPOOL

SPA' WATER,

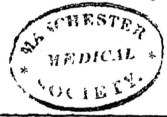

By THOMAS HOULSTON, M.D.

Mineral waters *often produce cures, which we in vain attempt to perform by the combinations in our shops; even altho' these waters contain nothing but* IRON.

Cullen's Lectures on the Materia Medica, p. 190.

LIVERPOOL:
Printed for A. WILLIAMSON, near the Exchange.
M,DCC,LXXIII.

PREFACE.

THE Spring which has been difcovered in the Stone Quarry on the fouth fide of Liverpool, having been much talked of, and ufed by many with evident advantage, I thought it might not be improper to endeavour at afcertaining its component principles, and, thence deducing its probable medical virtues. Convinced, both by reafon and experiment, that it promis'd no inconfiderable means of reftoring and preferving health, I fhould have accufed myfelf of inattention to the interefts of humanity, and to the welfare of fociety, had I not ufed my beft endeavours to promote and extend its ufe amongft my fellow citizens.

But what more particularly induced me to aim at recommending it to their notice, by this little publication, was the undoubted evidence I had collected of its having been of fignal fervice, even in fome defperate cafes : fome of thefe I have herein given, as the foundation of that confidence which I hope it may merit and obtain   Many mineral fprings, both in England and abroad, poffefs'd of the like properties

and

P R E F A C E.

and principles, have acquired the higheft reputation for their medicinal qualities and the cures
they have wrought.

I would not wifh to lay too great a ftrefs upon the virtues of our Liverpool Spà, but rather,
by afcribing to it fimply thofe it poffeffes, and
relating briefly and intelligibly fome of the cafes
in which it has been found greatly beneficial,
ftrive to excite the public to make a trial, which
may at once procure reputation to the fountain,
health to thofe who frequent it, and a heartfelt
fatisfaction to the propofer and promoter of it.

Liverpool, May 4th, 1773.

ESSAY

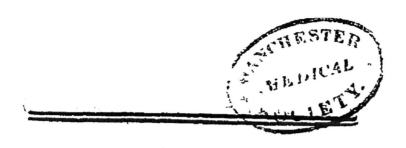

E S S A Y

On the LIVERPOOL SPA' WATER.

§ 1. Of MINERAL WATERS in general.

WE diftinguifh by the term of *mineral wa-ters*, thofe which are impregnated with fome *mineral* principles, and hence are become *medicinal*.

They are properly divided into SALINE, SUL-PHUREOUS, and METALLIC.

We have found that thofe which have been termed *Spirituous* are indebted for that title, to a *gas*, or fix'd air only, to which they owe their fparkling, and that agreeable, pungent, acidulous tafte, by which they refemble Champain. From this fame principal they acquire the property they poffefs of diffolving metallic fubftances, as will be fhewn hereafter. The peculiar acidulous tafte which it imparts, has occafioned their be-ing made, by fome, a feparate clafs under that denomination (Acidulæ) but, as it will appear,

that

that there are no waters abounding with fix'd air
which are not impregnated with other (mineral)
substances, and as few instances can be produced, in which an acid uncombin'd is found, in
any sensible proportion, in mineral waters, these
distinctions seem superfluous, if not improper.
The only instance I have seen of a mineral water really and abundantly containing an uncombined acid, is in a spring near Naples, call'd the
Pisciarelli, where the water issues out very hot
from the side of a volcano, and so acid as readily to corrode the surface of metals. But the
acidulous taste depending on this fix'd air is met
with even in waters, in which an alcali, uncombin'd, is found; as in the waters of St. Martin,
in Roussillon, and La Marquise, in Dauphiny.

Many mineral waters in all the classes possess
this fix'd air. The Seltzer water abounds
with it, and is little impregnated with any
other active principle; and hence the Seltzer
water may be easily imitated by a very small
addition of sea-salt and alcali to water saturated with fix'd air, separated, collected, and
applied after the manner of the ingenious Dr.
PRIESTLEY.

This is done still easier, by the process in-
vented by that great French Chymist, VENEL,
of adding the acid of sea-salt, in proper proportion,

portion, to water in which a very fmall portion of alcali is diffolv'd. No vifible effervefcence enfues (the mixture being fo very dilute) but the fix'd air, as it feparates from the combination of the acid and alcali, is abforb'd by the water, and impregnates it fo, as to give with very little trouble, a tolerable imitation of, and fuccedaneum for, the Seltzer water.

But I will not dwell too much on thefe diftinctions: my intention is not to write on the nature of mineral waters, but to point out the properties and effects of our own. Hence I fhall only flightly treat of the different claffes, as far as is requifite to convey a clear general idea of the nature and varieties of mineral waters, as an introduction to the examining and comprehending our Liverpool Spà.——— And it may be ufeful in this place to obferve, that we muft not expect to find the feveral claffes wholly diftinct from each other; on the contrary, they are generally all more or lefs combin'd together, fo that moft commonly they can only be clafs'd from the principle which is found to predominate.

§ 2. Of Saline Waters.

STRICTLY speaking, perhaps, all the mineral waters might be termed *Saline*, as all containing more or less an alcaline, neutral, earthy, or metallic salt. But by this term we generally only understand waters, chiefly containing neutral and earthy salts in a sensible proportion, so as to prove purgative.—The waters impregnated only with selenites (i. e. vitriolic acid, and calcareous earth) which is the case with all our hard pump water, do not, I think, deserve to be considered as saline mineral waters; as instead of being improved by this admixture, they are rendered unfit even for most domestic uses. The good effects of Bristol water (which contains scarcely any other saline matter than selenites) are not to be attributed to its solid contents, but to the fix'd air it abounds with; which is also the case with respect to some other mineral waters, which, though they contain neutral salts, yet those are in too small proportion to answer any good purpose ——Water is impregnated with selenites by passing through gypseous earth and stones, consisting of selenites which are soluble in water.

An alcaline salt uncombined is rarely to be found in mineral waters, or when it is, its proportion

portion and effects are inconsiderable. The Tilbury, Clifton, and Seltzer waters, *Eau de la Marquise* in Dauphiny, and *St Jean's*, have been considered as alcaline. The waters of this class, (if possess'd of any particular virtues) must be of service in all complaints arising from acidity, and act as attenuant, diuretic, and aperitive. Boyle, however, denied the existence of this class of waters in England

The acids found combin'd in mineral waters are, the Vitriolic or Universal, and Marine or acid of sea salt The Nitrous is not found, nor do I believe, that the Volatile Vitriolic acid (uncombin'd at least) has ever been proved to exist in waters Authors have labour'd long to prove the presence and escape of this volatile acid, and to reconcile thus the proofs that these acidulous waters contain a predominant alcaline basis. I find Hoffman, though he could not account for this, rejecting the opinion of a volatile vitriolic acid—*De Element Aquarum mineralium recte dijudicand et examinand* p 138, § xi *Neque enim, quod primus omnium ego observavi, purum acidum in acidulis deliteret, sed omnes, quotquot sunt et dicuntur, in omnibus Europæ locis, sal alcali vehunt; ut potius alcalinæ dicendæ essent.*

The

The difcoveries which have within thefe few years been made, chiefly by our own countrymen, refpecting the nature and properties of fix'd air, have render'd this matter much eafier to comprehend, than it was to former writers. When we find (with the Hon. Mr. Cavendifh*) that fix'd air diffolves calcareous earth, and metals (with Mr. Lane*); that it gives a fubtile fpirit or gas, and a very acidulous tafte to water, without impregnating it with any acid (as appears from Mr. Henry's Experiments), and when we fee this air readily efcapes and depofits the earth or metal with which it was combin'd, we fhall foon be convinc'd that this is what former writers miftook for a volatile vitriolic acid. Thefe properties of fix'd air will clear up at once all the difficulties they labour'd under, account for the feeming inconfiftencies they ftrive to reconcile, and, probably, afford to future writers a much clearer and more eligible method of claffing mineral waters, particularly if it fhould appear, as has been before hinted, that the medical virtues of many of thefe (as well faline as metallic) depend, chiefly, if not totally, on this principle.

---

* Philofophical Tranfact. 1765.
* Philofophical Tranfact. 1769.

But

But leaving this to thofe, who, *ex profeffo*, may hereafter take up the fubject of mineral waters, I fhall proceed with the combinations of the vitriolic and marine acid found therein; the moft frequent of which is the latter.

The waters of the fea, and of falt fprings, contain chiefly the marine acid, united with a mineral alcali, forming common falt, the ufes of which, both domeftic and medicinal, are confiderable. Authors account for this impregnation from the immenfe rocks of foffil falt found in various parts of the globe, of which we have no inconfiderable fpecimens in our own neighbourhood.

The waters of this clafs are known by their falt tafte. Some of the falt fprings are nearly pure, and contain little elfe but pure falt, as the upper pit at Droitwich Others are not free from earthy, and even metallic, mixtures, as thofe of Northwich in Chefhire, which contain fome portion of Magnefia, Calcareous earth, and iron. The brine pits at Droitwich yield little earth and no bittern; the reft do, and from this bittern a bitter purging falt is obtained, to which we have given the name of Epfom falt, and which is Magnefia combin'd with vitriolic acid. 'Tis this falt (refembling Glau-

ber's

ter's falt) on which depends the purgative quality of our several mineral waters, as those of
Epsom, Cheltenham, Acton, Scarborough, Har-
tlepool, Seltzer (or Seidlitz) &c. A small proportion of calcareous earth, of an oily sub-
stance, and in some, a very little iron, make the
rest of the substances which these waters are
found to contain.

As well as the S E A W A T E R.

The proportions are various in the different
waters. A pint of Epsom water contains about
33 grains of the purgative salt, and 6 of calcareous earth. Cheltenham, 46 grains of this salt,
and 22 of calcareous earth, with about half a
grain of iron (Ochre) Scarborough water contains nearly the same proportions as Epsom, but
with a small quantity of iron and fix'd air. The
purgative quality of sea water however, does not
depend wholly on the quantity of this bitter
earthy salt contain'd in it, for common salt alone,
in sufficient dose, proves purgative. The whole
of the two salts contain'd in a pint of our *sea
water* is about five drachms, and a pint, a pint
and a half, or a quart, is found necessary in
different habits to act as a purgative.

All our salt springs are so much impregnated
with saline substances, as makes it necessary to
dilute them to render them tolerably agreeable

to the ftomach, particularly, as the more the folution of thefe falts is dilute, the milder and furer is their operation.

The proportions in thefe fprings alfo are various The brine pit at Nantwich yields $\frac{1}{7}$, at Middlewich $\frac{1}{4}$, the ftrongeft at Droitwich $\frac{3}{8}$, the weaker, $\frac{1}{4}$ part of common efculent falt, befides the Epfom falt (fo call'd) which remains in the bittern.

As a fubftitute for the faline waters of Epfom, Cheltenham, &c. we may diffolve Epfom or Glauber's falt in water, in the proportion of half an ounce to a pint But it is obferved by Hoffman, Rutty, &c that the effects of the falt fo rediffolved, are not above half what would have been produced, by fuch a dofe of the water itfelf as contains that quantity of falt, and that thefe waters when boil'd to the confumption of half, are not proportionably increafed in ftrength.

Where the fea water can be procured, it anfwers in general all the intentions of the waters of this clafs.

U S E S.

Thefe faline waters are ufed either as alteratives or purgatives. They are attenuant, refolv-

ent,

ent, cooling, aperient, and diuretic. They are
beneficial in viscid foulnesses of the stomach and
intestines, cleansing and stimulating, and hence
frequently amend loss of appetite and of the
digestive faculty, and stop vomiting; in habitu-
al costiveness, pains of the stomach, heart-burn,
colics; in removing obstructions of the abdo-
minal viscera, as of the liver, spleen, &c. and
principally in jaundice arising from this cause
in promoting the menstrual and hæmorrhoidal
discharges, in hysteric and hypochondriac affections; in vertigo and head-ache proceeding
from a foul stomach, and in the epilepsy In a
sufficient dose they are excellent purgatives; they
leave no constipation after their action, nor do
they heat during it They are peculiarly adapted therefore, as a cooling purgative in inflammatory and cutaneous diseases. They destroy
worms by evacuating the mucus in which they
live and generate, and by which they are defended against the action of vermifuge medicines.
These waters are extolled by Musgrave in the
gout, and by Russel, Rutty, and other authors,
in a variety of obstinate chronic cases.

U N F I T.
They are improper in weak, delicate, habits,
for persons advanced in years, for such as have
weak breasts, diseas'd lungs, confirm'd tumours
of

of the vifcera, or acrid juices; and hence in
fcurvy, ftrangury, dropfy, convulfive afthma,
or afthma from water in the cheft.

Great good effects are alfo experienc'd from
their ufe *externally*——So much has been wrote
in praife of *fea bathing*, that I fhall fay little on
that head, as its efficacy in preferving health and
ftrength is generally known and confefs'd. It
will be found to coincide, in its effects, with
thofe of our Spá Water.

Nor is its efficacy only to be deduced, as being a *cold bath*. The falt, befides adding to its
gravity, has been thought to be beneficial as a
topical application. Hippocrates thought it in
many cafes more efficacious *warm*, as in contrac-
tions, indolent tumors, paralytic and dropfical
affections. Fortunately we are fo fituated, as to
enjoy very defirable conveniences for fea bathing
both cold and hot, * and it is to be hoped, that
fuch facility will by no means caufe us to defpife

---

* A *hot* falt water Bath is at any time prepared at our baths, on
giving an hours notice, an advantage this, which fhould not be con-
fined to cafes in which *falt water* may be thought ferviceable, as it is
certain great good effects may be expected in many complaints from
the ufe of a *warm bath* ——I am entirely of opinion with the ingenious Dr. Percival, that we do not, in England, confider warm bathing as highly, or ufe it as frequently, as it deferves. Abroad, much
benefit is both expected and experienced, from its more frequent ufe
in difeafes.

and

and neglect a powerful means of preserving and restoring health, which others, at a distance from such conveniences, know how to set a proper value on, and are at considerable pains to come and partake of.

---

§ 3. Of Sulphureous Waters.

THESE are impregnated with the liver of sulphur (i. e. sulphur combin'd with a mineral alcali, or a calcareous earth, and thus rendered soluble in water) and are easily distinguished by their fœtid smell, and disagreeable taste, resembling rotten eggs.

Of this class are those of Harrowgate, Moffat, Aix la Chapelle, of D'ax, Bourbon, Mont d'or, St. Amant, Bareges, Bonnes, Cauterets, Chaudes, Arles, and Alais in France, of Swadlingbar, of Baden in Lower Austria, of the Geronster at Spà, of la Solforata and some others near Rome, and several I have met with in Germany and Italy. The vapors from these waters blacken silver, and heighten the colour of gold, some of them almost instantaneously on exposure. Some are pellucid, others of a milky colour; but they deposit a whitish cloud on the addition of an acid. On their surface a gold co-colour'd, beautifully variegated, pellicle is observed.

The

The fulphureous waters may be imitated not unaptly, by adding to a drachm of the flowers of fulphur, a grain of lime or calcin'd magnefia, or fix grains of falt of tartar, rubbing them together, and infufing them in a quart bottle, not quite filled with water, for eight or ten hours in a gentle heat; or by boiling an ounce of fulphur in twelve pints of frefh made lime-water. The dofe of thefe is from three to four Pints.

We have three fulphureous [faline] waters in Lancafhire · 1ft Maudfley near Prefton, which is blue, intolerably fœtid, and contains 930 grains of common falt in a gallon: 2d. Braughton, between Skipton and Coln, of a whitifh colour, the gallon yielding three drachms of falt. and 3d Cickle Spà, a Mile from Braughton, which is clear, very fœtid, and contains 308 grains of falt in a gallon. From the quantity of falt contain'd, they all prove purgative.

U S E S.

The waters of this clafs invigorate, lightly affect the head on being firft drank, and generally infpire gaiety and chearfulnefs, which are fometimes followed by drowfinefs, they raife the fpirits and promote an appetite. They attenuate, ftimulate and cleanfe, promoting digeftion, perfpiration and the regular natural difcharges, and

C   hence

hence are ufeful in that variety of complaints which arife, from indigeftion, acidities, foulneffes, &c, to perfons in whom the circulation is flow and languid, and where there is laxity of the folids, debility of the ftomach, or acrimory in the fift paffages. Hence, alfo, they are recommended in obftructions of the vifcera, or of the glares, in cold defluxions, conftipation, to deftroy worms, and to cure intermittents; in fuppreffion of the menftrual and hæmorrhoidal difcharges, in melancholic, hypochondriac and hyfteric cafes, in cachexy, dropfy, fcurvy, fcrophula, gout, ftone, palfy and nervous affections. In external complaints, as in foul ulcers, cutaneous eruptions, tetters, the itch, and in retroceffion of cutaneous eruptions, they are much extolled.

After their ufe, if they have left the body in a relaxed ftate, it may be neceffary to have recourfe to cold bathing and ftrengthening remedies, fuch as bark, &c. in order to reftore the tone of the fibres.

U N F I T.

They are improper in inflammatory and very irritable habits, in bilious, hectic, and feverifh complaints, in ulcers, tubercles, or infarctions of the lungs, in convulfive coughs and violent afthma

afthma from extravafated fluids, and in a dif-
pofition to Hæmorrhage and apoplexy.

We come now to the third and laft clafs of
Mineral waters, viz. the *Metallic*.

---

§ 4. Of Metallic Waters.

THESE have been fometimes ftiled *Vitriolic*,
as being all impregnated with a metallic
fubftance diffolv'd in the vitriolic or univerfal
acid. But thofe who have adopted this term
were unacquainted with the folvent property of
fix'd air. However, the vitriolic is the acid
moft frequently found in metallic waters, aud
is therein combin'd with zinc, copper or iron,
Water is impregnated with thefe principles by
meeting, in its paffage, with Pyrites (or Fire-
ftone) in a ftate of decompofition. The particular metal will depend on the nature of the
Pyrites.

The combination with zinc is rarely met
with ; — that with copper not frequently, and
as thefe have not been regarded as medicinal, it
fuffices fimply to have enumerated them. The

waters

waters of Neufol in Hungary, of two fprings
in the county of Wicklow in Ireland, and of one
in the Ifle of Anglefey, contain the vitriol of
copper. The copper is obtained from them
for fale, by adding to them iron : this is diffolv'd by the vitriolic acid, which deferts the
copper, and fuffers it to precipitate.,

But no impregnation is more frequently found
in mineral waters than that of iron, either diffolv'd by the vitriolic acid, or by means of fix'd
air, which has been generally confider'd as volatile vitriolic acid. Thefe waters, to which we
give the names of Martial, Ferrugineous, or Chalybeate (the latter very improperly, as fteel, i. e.
chalybs, is not a natural, but an artificial produc-
tion) are eafily known by their aftringent, ftyptic, tafte, and by leaving on the ftones, &c.
thro' which they run, a reddifh or ruft-like
ochre But if they be added to any aftringent
vegetable juice, as the infufion of tea, galls,
&c. they betray at once their nature by ftriking
a black, inky, colour.

Iron, is at once the hardeft, moft common,
ufeful, perfectly innocent, and eafily foluble,
of all the metals. And hence we need not
wonder at the number of mineral waters of
this clafs which are in high repute, fuch as
thofe

thofe of Pyrmont, Spá, Malmendy, Bath, Tunbridge, Hampftead, Iflington, Carlfbadt, Cleves, of Paffy in France, of Schwalbach in Heffe, of Freyenwald near Berlin, and many others.

In fome of thefe the iron is diffolv'd by the vitriolic acid, in others by fix'd air, and in many partly by each of thefe. The latter waters are fuch as, on ftanding, or boiling, precipitate an ocre, yet ftill retain, though in a lefs degree, the aftringent, ftyptic, tafte, and the property of ftriking black with galls. But it is remarkable that fo very fmall a proportion of martial vitriol, as one grain in a gallon of water, is fufficient to produce the change of colour with galls to a darkifh blue.

Waters ftrongly-impregnated with the vitriol of iron are not frequently met with, but thofe of Rammelfberg in Hungary, are confiderably fo. Such, however, are not fit for medical ufes.

The waters of this clafs might be imitated by diffolving a proper, fmall, proportion of the vitriol of iron in pure water. I fay, *fmall* proportion, becaufe there feems reafon for afcribing the good effects of martial waters, to the iron being thus adminifter'd in repeated fmall dofes.

But

But as we are at no lofs for chalybeate waters, and as nature is far more perfect in her combinations than we can be, it will rarely be neceffary to imitate her in this.

U S E S.

The effects are, thofe of iron in general, which we fhall referve for the next article.

2 Iron is diffolved in mineral waters, alfo by means of fix'd air, without the intervention of any acid. This, which is only a late difcovery, has formerly been the occafion of much perplexity, and authors finding fome chalybeate waters evincing marks of a predominant alcali, have endeavour'd to account for this feeming contradiction by ingenious fictions, of a *volatile vitriol*, or (with fomewhat lefs abfurdity) by fuppofing them to contain iron diffolv'd by means of the volatile vitriolic acid, which, on expofure to air, or heat, flying off, left the iron and fuffered it to precipitate. Pity it is, that fyftems fhould not only be fram'd, but for a fucceffion of years implicitly adopted, which have never undergone the teft of experiment, and which, by one of the moft fimple and obvious might eafily have been confuted. Unfortunately for this fyftem, it appears by experiment, that iron, when diffolv'd by means of

volatile

volatile vitriolic acid, will bear not only expofure to the air, but even a boiling heat without
either the vitriol or the acid totally flying off.
And where iron is diffolv'd by the fix'd air only, the air when at liberty foon flies off, the iron
(in ochre) precipitates, and the water no longer
ftrikes a black colour with the vegetable aftrin-
gents.

Many chalybeate waters (even fuch as contain iron diffolv'd in an acid) contain the iron
alfo diffolv'd by means of fix'd air, as thofe of
Spá, Pyrmont, Tunbridge, Bath, Cheltenham,
&c. And fuch as contain no iron, but only
fix'd air, as thofe of Buxton, Pifa, Seltzer, &c.
are found readily to diffolve iron filings, tho'
they evidently contain no acid.

By this means, or, by impregnating water with
fix'd air, after the manner of Doctor Prieftley,
we can imitate perfectly well, the Chalybeate
waters of this clafs.

U S E S.

Of the latter chalybeates, fome of the medical virtues are to be deduced from the action of
the *fix'd air* contain'd in them. This warms,
exhilarates, invigorates, reftores appetite, good
digeftion, proper circulation, and neceffary fe-
cretions.

cretions   It removes obftructions arifing from
a languid circulation, and reftores to the fibres
their tone and elafticity.   It is an excellent fti-
mulus, and a powerful corrector of any putrid
tendency.   From its active, fubtil, penetrating
nature, much may be expected, in hyfteric, hypochondriac, and nervous habits, in the rheu-
matifm, gout, palfy, and in many confumptive
cafes.—But from the *metallic principle* contain'd
in the waters of this clafs (of which we fhall
demonftrate the Liverpool Spá to be one) confiderable good effects may be expected.

Iron is aftringent, and antifpafmodic in fmall
dofes, it is tonic and ftrengthening, acting upon
the fibres and veffels of the ftomach and intef-
tines, and hence is excellent in difeafes caus'd
by laxity, debility, and inactivity of the digeftive organs, fuch as crudities, bad digeftion,
accompanied with flatulence, colics, fluxes, &c.
in cafe of general laxity and debility, and in hy-
fterics, unlefs there be invincible obftructions of
the vifcera, in intermittents, in the fcurvy, in
obftruction, and defect of fecretion and excretion caus'd by weaknefs and relaxation of the
fibres, as in rickets, fcrophula, chlorofis, fome
kinds of jaundice, &c. It fpeedily remedies lofs
of appetite, ftrengthens the ftomach and intef-
tines, deftroys worms, and cures obftructed
menftrua.

menftrua. But it muft be remembered, that this
change of the tone, and fpring of the
folids, cannot be effected but by a continuance
of the martial remedy, in fmall dofes, for fome
confiderable time, otherwife only a temporary
relief will enfue.

Some of thefe vitriolic waters are good to
ftop Hæmorrhages, particularly one at Haigh
in Lancafhire, one gallon of which is found to
contain 1920 grains of white and green vitriol.

U N F I T.

Wherever there is rigidity of the folids, an
increas'd impetus of the fluids, plethora, or a dif-
pofition to inflammation, this medicine is improper. In hectic fevers with a fpitting of blood,
it is little to be relied on, as, by encreafing the
tone, it may eafily encreafe both the fever and
hæmoptoe.

---

§ 5. On the Liverpool SPA'.

THIS water fprings, or ouzes, through veins
of that foft yellow ftone generally ufed
here for building and which owes its colour to
the iron which it contains. This ftone hardens in

the

the air, and when calcin'd, is of a red colour.
There are feveral fprings in this quarry, though
fituated very high, but none fo much impregnated as the one reforted to. * The water
trickles flowly into an irregular bafon (which
might be much enlarged) containing about four
gallons. It is naturally limpid, tho' frequently
found otherwife, owing to the ochre, which it
depofits on the efcape of the fix'd air, and as it
is expofed to the air and weather exhibits different appearances, and different proportions of
mineral contents, at different times. Its tafte is
at firft cool and refrefhing, afterwards auftere
and inky, and it does not lofe the irony tafte by
long keeping in open veffels, though it foon
depofits a quantity of ochre. Some time after
it has been drank, it is found by many to warm
the ftomach, and fome think they experience
from it, both a cordial, and lightly inebrieting,
fenfation. It has no fmell, and will keep a long
time without putrefying. It is one of thofe chalybeates which lofe leaft by keeping, and that
part of the iron which fubfides is fo minutely
divided, that, if fwallowed, it is readily re-dif-
folved in the ftomach. To inveftigate more
fully the nature and contents of this water, I
fubmitted it to the following Experiments.

---

* A fmaller one near it is ufed for external applications, to wafh
the eyes, ulcers, &c, and contains iron, but in fmaller proportion.

EXPE-

EXPERIMENT I.

A glafs of the Liverpool Spá Water expofed
to the air for 24 hours, depofited a quantity of
an ochrous earth, which, on adding an acid, rediffolved perfectly.   The fame thing happened,
but in a fhorter time, by placing a glafs of this
water in a moderate degree of heat (a water
bath) a number of air bubbles, and a depofition
of ochre followed in a fhort time.   This depofition was effected ftill fooner by boiling.

This experiment feems to prove, that a portion of the iron contain'd in this water is kept
in a ftate of folution, by means of *fix'd air*, the
efcape of which being permitted by expofure
in open veffels, or promoted by expofure to
heat, the iron fo diffolved is foon precipitated.
That the whole, however, of the iron contain'd
is not diffolved by *fix'd air*, appears from the
following experiments.

EXPERIMENT II.

To the water boil'd, a little tea, or a few
drops of the infufion of galls being added, gave
a blackifh purple colour ; to that which had
ftood fome hours in the water bath, a much
deeper, for the black colour produced in
this, from the above additions, was nearly
equal to what appeared on their mixture

D 2   with

with the water which had only been expofed to
the air. The ir'ty colour is in all much heightened by ftanding, and the more fo, when the
water is frefh taken from the fpring, and when
not diluted by accidental circumftances. This
water, there ore, will always contain a greater
proportion of the metallic principle in a ftate
of folution, the frefher it is drank.

E X P E R I M E N T   III.

Fix'd alcali (pot afh) added to fome of the
water boil'd an hour, caufed a fmall quantity of
ochre to precipitate, from the water expofed to
a moderate heat, a greater quantity, from that
expofed to the air only 14 days, ftill more; and
from the frefh water immediately a confiderable
portion was feparated. Hence 'tis plain that
befides her diffolved by means of a volatile folvent, this water contains alfo that metal diffolv'd
in an acid, from which it is readily feparated by
the addition of an alcaline falt, which has a
greater attraction, or affinity, to acids, than metals have.

E X P E R I M E N T   IV.

A gallon of the water collected foon after a
heavy rain, and which feem'd weaker than ordinary, both to the tafte, and to other trials,

was

was fuffer'd to remain in open veffels, till it had
depofited its ochre, which, when feparated by
filtering, weigh'd four grains· It was then evaporated in a glafs veffel with a gentle fire, and
when reduced to a fourth part, was filter'd a-
gain, four grains of ochre remain'd in the filtre,
yet the clear liquor proved, on the addition of
galls, &c. that it ftill retain'd a portion of iron.

EXPERIMENT V.

The *fame* water, evaporated to half a pint
and filtred, was of a reddifh colour, and ftruck
black with galls. The remaining part of the
evaporation was made in a water bath, and as it
proceeded, a quantity of falt kept rifing to the
furface, forming a fhining pellicle, and fubfiding.
When reduced to about two ounces and cool, it
was examined in the microfcope, and * chryftals,
refembling needles, were obferved ranging themfelves into a ftar-like form. The laft drop of
fluid remaining, examin'd in like manner, gave
cubical chryftals The whole had, towards
the end of the evaporation, a greenifh colour,
and vitriolic fmell, and fome of the chryftals
which had form'd on the fides of the veffel

* Nice Microfcopical Obfervations on the different forms of chryf-
tallizing falts, might probably contribute not a little to the readily
diftinguifhing the different kinds, and thus affift both analyzation and
metallurgy · at leaft, this fubject offers a fcope for highly curious and
entertaining experiments.

deliquefced

deliquefced (i. e. abforbing moifture from the air, re-diffolv'd)—The quantity of folid contents were,

Of ochre which fubfided, four grains;

Of ochre feparated by boiling and filtring, four grains;

Remaining when evaporated to drynefs, twenty grains;--- in all 28 grains; whereas the total of folid contents in a gallon of Tunbridge water is only nine grains, and fometimes much lefs; and of the Geronfter at Spà, 24 grains. (Rutty)

EXPERIMENT VI.

The whole of the folid contents remaining on evaporating to drynefs, were wafhed with hot water, as long as they yielded any faline impregnation to it. The filtred liquor, at firft was of a deep amber colour, inclining to green, and ftruck black immediately with galls. It did not fuffer any fenfible alteration with acids, nor make any immediate change in the colour of fyrup of violets, but an alcali precipitated from it a green powder, and in fhort it gave, on every trial, undoubted marks of its containing martial vitriol (or iron diffolv'd in the vitriolic acid) and that in fuch proportion, as, I believe, would juftify my afferting the Liverpool Spà, to be one of the moft powerful, pure, and perfect chaly-

beates,

beates, in ufe, in England; not liable, as many
are, to lofe its virtue by keeping.

EXPERIMENT VII.

The water in which the falts were rediffolved,
as in the laft experiment, was again evaporated;
and the falts chryftallized, nearly in the fame
order as before. Thofe which chryftallized
firft, ftruck a much deeper black with galls,
than thofe which formed only towards the end
of the evaporation. There had remained in the
filtre, a fine grey powder, which did not effervefce
with acids, and turned black on a hot iron. This
weighed one grain---Of the falts much the
greater part was martial vitriol. They did not
effervefce with acids or alcalies fenfibly: on the
hot iron they fcarcely decrepitated, but turn'd
of a deep red colour, like colcothar, emitting
a flight fume. This calcin'd matter was moftly
infoluble in water, and alfo in acids, yet had a
faltifh tafte.

The other falts joined with the martial vitriol
in this water, are in fo fmall proportion, as to
merit but little attention in the analyfis, and
ftill lefs the enumeration of various experiments,
proving what they are not I have reafon to believe,
however, they confift of the marine acid, combin'd

bin'd firſt with iron, (deliquefcing) and fecondly, with magnefia, or calcareous earth.

EXPERIMENT VIII.

The Syrup of violets added to this water produced no immediate change of colour, * no more than the red juice of the rind of radiſhes, a proof that neither an acid nor an alcali un-combin'd, is contain'd in it, fince a drop of di-lute vitriolic acid caufed the mixture immediate-ly to turn a bright red, and a fmall portion of alcali rendered it green. Boil'd with milk, it does not coagulate it, but encreafes its fweet taſte : it lathers alfo with foap ; further proofs of its containing no uncombined acid. I think, however, I have obferved, on mixing the red juice of radiſhes with the water which had un-dergone a long evaporation in glafs veffels, and depofited much ochre, that the red colour was heightened, as if an acid then predominated.

---

* After ſtanding fome time it became of a fea green , but we muſt obferve that this change of the blue juices to a green, is effect-ed, not only by a predominant alcali, but alfo by the folutions of Iron, in the fix'd or volatile vitriolic acid, or in fix'd air —May not the want of attention to this circumſtance have given rife to confu-fion and miſtake on the fubject?

EXPERIMENT IX.

Cauftic volatile alcali was added to the Li-verpool Spà Water. An ochrous precipitation enfued, but no change of colour · a proof that it contains no copper, for if it did, a beautiful blue would have been produced on the mixture.

---

§ 6. REMARKS and EXPERIMENTS, on the VOLATILE SOLVENT.

WE have hitherto taken for granted, that the Volatile Solvent in Chalybeate waters, was fix'd air, and have poftponed, to the article of experiment, the reafons for denying it to be the volatile vitriolic acid, and for concluding it to be fix'd air. As this is a fubject which has as yet been little canvaffed, and as a contrary opinion is ftill maintained by men, whofe ingenuity, learning and reputation give weight to their theory, it feemed but juft, to confider this matter a little more minutely.

Till within thefe few years the nature and properties of fix'd air were little, if at all, underftood : and Mr Lane firft, in the year 1769, publifh'd to the world, that it was capable of

E   diffolving

diffolving iron. Before that time, as no other folvent, of a fugitive nature, was known, except volatile vitriolic acid, authors attributed to *it*, the folution of iron in fuch chalybeate waters, as, on ftanding a fhort time expofed to the air, depofite their metallic contents, and lofe their confequent virtues: and even later authors on this fubject have been fo far influenced by the authority, and prevailing opinion, of their predeceffors, as to adopt this concluſion without fufficient examination, or the fhadow of proof. For, in reality, the exiftence of this volatile acid in chalybeate waters has never yet been fairly proved by experiment, and perhaps will be found to be, the child of invention, adopted by neceffity, and foftered by ignorance of the truth.

The inconveniences and abfurdities derived from fupporting this theory are apparent in moft works on the fubject. We need look, for an inftance of it, no farther back, than in that elaborate author, Rutty, p. 325, on the waters of Spà, he writes thus · " they contain a good deal of air, and a volatile acid, difcoverable by the tafte,--and at the fame time,--an alcaline falt predominating over the acid, as is evident from the appearances exhibited, &c."

But

But a later very learned and ingenious writer, who, is well acquainted both with chemiftry in general, and with the doctrines relative to fix'd air, Dr. Falconer of Bath, though he proves the prefence of " fix'd air, in confiderable proportion," in the Bath waters, yet attributes the folution of iron therein, rather to volatile vitriolic acid, than to it. In his Effay on Bath Waters, p. 220. *2d Edition*, he gives an eafy method of afcertaining the prefence of the volatile acid, viz. by adding Magnefia, with which it effervefces. But this will by no means determine whether the iron be diffolved by volatile, or fixed vitriolic acid, as, in the preceding paragraph, we find this effervefcence propofed as a teft of the latter alfo.* Yet by his 16th. Experiment, it appears that Bath Waters did not thus effervefce. This then cannot amount to a certain proof of the volatile acid being the folvent, no more can the partial decompofition, and depofition of ochre on ftanding, as the fame thing happens alfo from a dilute folution of iron, in the fixed vitriolic acid.† A remark made by

* I apprehend here is fome miftake. With refpect to the volatile vitriolic acid, there certainly is, as the combination of that with Iron, however concentrated, caufes no fuch effervefcence. Neither does our Spa Water, nor a folution of martial vitriol in water.

† One grain of martial vitriol, diffolved in half a pint of water had a confiderable depofition on ftanding.

the

the Dr p. 186, feems to offer a means of deter-
mining the queftion, viz. that fixed air diffolves
iron and not copper, volatile vitriolic acid, diffolves both very plentifully. But in making
the experiment, an obfervation made by Dr. Percival, muft be remembered, " that the fixed
vitriolic acid when its falts are diluted, is fe-
perable and diffipated by a boiling heat."

The prefence of a volatile vitriolic acid being
by no means proved, it can only be faid to be
implied by analogy, or fupported by probability.
Let us fee then, if we fhall not find, even in the
Doctors Effay, reafons for afferting, that thefe
make in favour of fix'd air as the folvent. P.
294, he tells us that " Bath Water poured on
iron filings diffolves them plentifully; yet p.
261, that this water moft probably contains no
acid uncombined, or if any, not above a drop
in many pounds, and—that the vitriolic acid
does not remain in the water in its feperate
ftate " If fo, what does it contain capable of
diffolving the filings of iron plentifully, but the
fix'd air? The learned author allows, p. 186,
that the volatile vitriolic acid, though a poffible,
is, nothing near fo frequent an impregnation
(of mineral waters) as fix'd air.

For

For farther light on this subject, and to prove if possible, that the volatile vitriolic acid is not the solvent in such chalybeates as lose all their metallic impregnation, on a short exposure to the air, I procured about half an ounce of volatile vitriolic acid, by destilling in a sand heat, with the greatest care, in glass vessels, two ounces of vitriolic acid, from a little charcoal. It came over colourless, and scarcely acid to the taste, diffusing through the whole house a pungent, suffocating smell, like that of a burning match. It did not effervesce with the mildest alcalies, nor with Magnesia. Instead of changing the blue juices red, as it did before distillation, it deprived them, and the red flowers, of all colour, the mixture however became of a bright red, on standing 24 hours; this circumstance naturally suggested the following,

EXPERIMENT X.

A few drops of this volatile vitriolic acid, was diluted with an ounce of water, and suffered to remain in a glass open to the air, for 24 hours. The blue juice of the Iris was then added, and immediately changed to a bright red.

When this happened in the former experiment, it might be supposed, that the volatile acid was retained and fixed by the blue juices,

but

but in this no such detention is to be apprehended. We see then clearly, that *volatile vitriolic
acid*, when diluted, and *exposed* some time to the
air, instead of flying off, as was supposed, be-
comes *fixed*. How is it probable then, it should
so soon dissipate in mineral waters, wherein, be-
sides being in a like state of dilution, it is combined with, and retained by iron?

But the following experiment proves beyond
a doubt, that the volatile vitriolic acid is *not* the
solvent, in such chalybeates, as readily lose, on
exposure to the air, their metallic principles.

EXPERIMENT XI.

To a pint of spring water were added, ten
drops of the volatile vitriolic acid, which had
remained twenty hours on fresh filings of iron,
and which seemed fully saturated with the metal. The mixture struck a fine purple with
galls. One half of it was immediately boiled
on an open fire, in a Florence flask, for a quar-
ter of an hour and filtered, it then struck a deeper purple with galls than before, and continued
so to do when evaporated almost to dryness, after standing in a bason twenty one days. A
piece of paper dyed blue, and put in the neck
of the flask, had lost its colour, which did not
happen on the evaporation of our Spa Water.
The

The other half ſtood in a baſon twenty four hours, without ſcarcely any ochre ſubſiding, and, after remaining expoſed to the air about three weeks, ſtruck inſtantly black with galls. Its taſte was like that of our Spa Water, but a little ſulphureous.

EXPERIMENT XII.

A freſh mixture, of the ſolution of iron in the vol. vitriolic acid, with water, was evaporated to dryneſs by a gentle heat. The dry remainder conſiſted partly of ochre, and partly of a ſaline ſubſtance, which chryſtallized in a ſtar-like form in the microſcope, ſimilar to what we obſerve in a ſolution of iron, by the fixed vitriolic acid, when evaporated to dryneſs. The ſalt had an aſtringent taſte, turned black with galls, green with the blue juices, and precipitated an ochre on adding an alcali to the ſolution of it. Is it poſſible after this to ſuppoſe that a ſolution of iron in vol. vitriolic acid, is ſo readily and per-fectly decompoſed, by expoſure to the air, as hitherto has been taken for granted, or is it not rather clear, that 'tis as difficultly decompoſed, as that with the fix'd acid?

A remark made by Mr. Lane, coincides per-fectly with the above experiments, and, as ap-pears from thence, extends alſo to the volatile acid.

acid. Philos. Tranfact. 1769, page 222 —
" Where iron is fufpended in water by an acid,
" neither expofure nor boiling will deftroy its
" property of tinging with galls, which is the
" reverfe of what we find to be the cafe with
" many ferrugineous waters."

Of this nature is one in the neighbourhood of
Crofby (at Holmer Green, in Thornton) which
ftrikes inftantly a Burgundy colour with galls,
exactly fimilar to that, which a dilute folution
of iron by means of fix'd air produced. This
chalybeate, when kept three days, had loft all
its metallic impregnation, and with it, its power of tinging with galls. It is conftantly drank,
and ufed for all domeftic purpofes, by a very
healthy family, who prefer it to any pure water.
There is another of the fame kind near it, (at the
Lunt): both of thefe owe their metallic impregnation to fix'd air, as may be inferred from the
following,

EXPERIMENT XIII

Ten grains of iron filings ftood three days
in four ounces of water impregnated with fix'd
air. The iron was fcarcely diminifhed in weight,
but an ounce of this folution gave, to a pint of
fpring water, the tafte and properties of a chalybeate, fuch as the Crofby Spá; it ftruck the

fame

fame colour with galls, and, *like it*, when kept three days, loft this property entirely.

Fix'd air then is capable of diffolving iron, and that metal, fo diffolved, communicates to water, properties, evidently correfponding with thofe of the chalybeates which readily fpoil by keeping. Yet the following feems to prove, that fix'd air is not, in its nature, an acid, nor is any acid carried up into the water, during its impregnation with fix'd air.

EXPERIMENT XIV.

Four ounces of water were faturated with fix'd air, and obtained an acidulous tafte, yet did not, even on ftanding, make the leaft change in the colour of fyrup of violets, nor of the juice of the Iris, though that is one of the beft tefts of an acid Nor could I, by transfufing, for a long time, fix'd air feparated from a mixture of chalk and vitriolic acid, into water dyed blue, produce the leaft change in the colour towards a red. On the contrary, the blue colour was difcharged, a bluifh fediment formed, and the water became entirely colourlefs. The fix'd air, herein, feemed to poffefs the property of volatile vitriolic acid, of deftroying the colour of flowers, for a piece of the blue Iris, infufed

F

in the water impregnated as above, was deprived of its colour, without communicating any
tinge to the water.

Dr. Falconer, in his Effay, p. 314, admits
that " fix'd air changes to a red colour the blue
juices, and that it is not improbable, that an
acid is always either united with, or makes part
of, the compofition of fix'd air." But does
not his experiment, p. 143, of fix'd air diffolving iron diffufed through a folution of mild alcali, prove the contrary.

Having, I hope, proved, that volatile vitriolic acid *can not* be the folvent, in fugitive chalybeates, and offered reafons, and experiments
in fupport of fix'd air being the folvent, we
fhould now, apply this to our Liverpool Spà,
and, if poffible, bring proof of the exiftence
of this principle therein. But it may perhaps,
not be fo eafy to collect pofitive proofs of it;
firft, becaufe, from the nature of its fituation,
the greateft part of its fix'd air muft efcape, whilft the water trickles down the
fide of the rock, which is, hence, cover'd
thick with the ochre depofited, and whilft it remains quite open to the air : fecondly, becaufe
it is naturally contained therein, in very fmall
proportion united with the iron. We found
by

by experiment 13th, how very fmall a proportion of iron diffolv'd by fix'd air, was fufficient to imitate a chalybeate water of the fugitive kind. A ftill lefs proportion may be expected in waters, which are befides impregnated with martial vitriol. Thefe circumftances render it difficult to collect the fix'd air in fufficient quantity, fo as to prove indubitably its exiftence by any experiment.—Let us fee how far analogy and probability will affift in fupporting this pofition.

Mr. Worthington, in his experiments on the Liverpool Spà, publifh'd during the printing of thefe fheets (by which I find we were both employed on the fame fubject, unknown to each other) gives up, feemingly with reluctance, the opinion of fix'd air, being the folvent of a part of the iron in this water. Yet the following paffages, in his work, feem to corroborate the truth of it. P. 14, he makes this ingenious remark " the colour of the water is altered, from the greater or leffer degree of elafticity in the air, the more elaftic, the brighter, and from the want of elafticity, the more opaque." It is certain, that when the air is moft elaftic, it will moft powerfully counteract and impede the diffipation of the fix'd air, which keeps part of the iron in a ftate of folution, on the contrary, when the air is lefs elaftic, the fix'd air, being

more

more at liberty, will fooner fly off, and the o-
chre precipitate, and occafion the water to become turbid. But it by no means appears that
this would be the cafe if the iron was diffolved
by the volatile vitriolic acid ; fee experiments
11, 12.—How otherwife than by diffipating
the fix'd air, can " the funs influence impair its
virtues, or injure its qualities, by a partial decompofition," as he obferves it does, p. 15, 24.
I have before explained the difficulties which
oppofe themfelves to our attempts to demonftrate, by experiment, the exiftence of fix'd air
in the water. Hence 'tis no wonder if Mr.
Worthington's experiment with lime water, did
not fucceed to prove it. The German Spá, and
fome other of the like chalybeates, contain not
only fix'd air in union with iron, but a fuper-
abundance of fix'd air uncombined, thefe waters fpring out in large quantity, and proper
fteps are taken to prevent the evaporation of
this volatile principle, and hence, we find them
exhibit fenfible proofs of their containing fix'd
air. But Mr. W. admits that the Liverpool
Spà, though without thefe advantages, contains " an extraordinary quantity of common air
exceedingly elaftic, fo as, when held before the
fire, to force the cork, with fome explofion,
out of a vial three fourths filled." What common water, equally expofed, contains fo great

a quantity? A ftrong prefumptive proof in favour of our argument might be deduced from his 13th experiment, p 20, where " fix'd or mephitic air transfufed, reftored the fpoiled water," by rediffolving the ochre precipitated on expofure to the air, and by this means, as we find p 22, it " recovered its qualities more perfectly than by the addition of vitriolic acid," had not Mr. Lane, in the Philof. Tranfactions, 1769. Exp 2 p 218, tried in vain to rediffolve by means of fix'd air, the ochre precipitated; which was foluble in the vitriolic acid, and if, on repeating the experiment, I had not been equally unfuccefsful. For I find, not only fix'd air does not rediffolve the whole of the ochre precipitated, but that neither the volatile vitriolic, nor marine acid, does it other than in part. But tho' fix'd air does not perfectly rediffolve the ochre, yet it certainly does in part, for the fpoiled water, which before gave only a faint blackifh tinge with galls, when impregnated with fix'd air, gave, in the fame proportions, a beautiful purple colour. Does not this feem as if we reftored to it its properties, by replacing what it had loft on expofure?

The following may perhaps be deemed not unworthy a place here as a prefumptive argument in favour of fix'd air, one of the principle pro-

perties

perties of which is, its refifting and correcting
the putrefaction of animal fubftances.

EXPERIMENT XV.

A bit of the lean of lamb, in weight half a
drachm, was put into a phial, clofe cork'd, with
two ounces of the frefh Spa Water; a like piece
was put into an open veffel, with the fame quantity of Spa Water; a third, into two ounces of
our beft pump water; and all three were placed
in a warm room   In 48 hours, that in pump
water, began to acquire a putrid fmell, and in
four days became quite fœtid   Four days were
compleated, before that in Spà Water expofed
to the air became offenfive; the fibres feem'd
corrugated, and there was a fhining fcum on the
furface: in two days more, it was to the full as
fœtid as the former.   That clofe corked, open'd
the 10th. day, was fcarcely offenfive, nor rofe
to the furface: the 13th day, the bottle was
broke by accident, the meat was by no means
putrid, but rather harder than when frefh, and
infufed in frefh Spà Water, open to the air,
did not become putrid till four days more were
expired   It would feem then, that this water
refifts putrefaction, and the more powerfully,
when the efcape of the fix'd air is prevented.

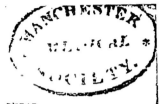

E X P E R I M E N T   XVI.

A phial containing five grains of the bright filings of iron, was filled with four ounces of the fresheft Liverpool Spâ Water, close corked, and kept with the mouth downwards, two days. The iron vifibly attracted bubbles of air, and with them, particles of it were carried up to the furface. The water was then filtered and ftruck with galls, a much deeper purple than the fresh Spa Water did; the iron remaining in the filtre, did not feem to be at all diminifhed in weight, when accurately examined; in this refpect refembling Antimony which gives a ftrong impregnation to wine, in which it is infufed, without fuffering any fenfible diminution.

We have already feen that this water contains no acid uncombined, and hence we can only attribute the folution and additional impregnation, to the action of that fmall portion of fix'd air uncombined, which remains in the water, upon the iron. Is not this then a ftronger prefumptive proof in favour of fix'd air, than any which has been advanced in favour of volatile vitriolic acid ?

E X P E R I M E N T   XVII.

In a former experiment, [13] fix'd air combin'd with iron, was found to produce a burgundy colour,

lour with galls, and there is reafon to believe that chalybeate waters give a reddifh tinge in proportion as they contain fix'd air, whereas vol vitriolic acid and iron gave a blackifh tinge. The following, are the appearances produced by the addition of a grain of powdered galls, to two ounces of each of thefe waters.

Frefh Crofby Spà Water; ⎰ a Burgundy co-
Artificial fix'd air chalybeate, ⎱ lour immediately.

Thefe, when expofed 3 days, ⎰ no change of colour
⎱

Artificial vol. vitriolic chaly- ⎰ immediately
beate, after ftanding 14 days, ⎱ blackifh.

Liverpool Spá Water, ditto ⎱ a blackifh purple.

Do.   frefh   ⎰ at firft, a Burgundy
⎱ or claret.

Do. which had ftood two ⎰ a much deeper claret
days on iron,   ⎱

    Thefe became purple with a reddifh caft.

Do. which had remain'd 4 ⎰ on ftanding, a beau-
days on iron,   ⎱ tiful deep purple.

Do. kept four days corked, ⎱
in a cool room, but had let ⎰ on ftanding, a faint
fall part of its iron,   ⎱ blackifh fhade.

Do. Do. with the addition ⎰ a good purple with
of fix'd air,   ⎱ a reddifh caft.

EXPERIMENT XVIII.

To have produced a pofitive, uncontroverti-
ble proof of the prefence of fix'd air, we fhould
have fhewn, that the vapor of the Spa Water
fuffices to reftore to a cauftic alcali, the fix'd
air of which it had been deprived by the addition of lime. But the circumftances which render the detention of the fix'd air fo difficult,
have been already explained, and hence I need
not fcruple to avow, that I have more than once
unfuccefsfully tried the following experiment.
A bent tube was paffed through the cork of a
quart bottle, carefully filled at the Spà early in
the morning; the other end of it was inferted
into a phial, containing cauftic fix'd alcali, and
the bottle after ftanding fome time before the
fire was put into a water bath; but I have not
yet been lucky enough, by this means, to reftore
to the alcali, its faculty of effervefcing with an
acid, though it became turbid, and a partial
precipitation of the lime took place, which are
advances towards the ftate of a mild alcali,
and owing to a fmall quantity of fix'd air, tho'
not fufficient to faturate the alcali.

EXPERIMENT XIX.

Lime water, mix'd with an equal quantity of
frefh Spà Water, caufed a yellow ochrous precipitation; in confequence of the lime ab-

G   forbing

forbing the fix'd air, which is the folvent of part of the iron herein

But as I fear I have already trefpaffed upon the patience of many readers on this matter, however interefting it may appear to fome, I fhall here drop the fubject and proceed to,

---

§ 7. VIRTUES of the LIVERPOOL SPA' WATER.

THIS water then contains, beyond a doubt, iron diffolv'd, both by fix'd air, and by vitriolic acid : in this latter circumftance, having the advantage over Tunbridge, and moft of our other chalybeates. This renders it not liable, like them, to depofite its metallic principle by keeping Yet the martial vitriol is fo very much diluted and fo minutely divided, as to render it at once extremely beneficial, perfectly innocent, and adapted even to weak ftomachs. *

---

* They are a mild, native tincture of fteel, having this peculiar excellence that they agree with the moft tender fubjects even where fteel in fubftance is attended with ill effects, and by the extreme fubtility of their parts penetrate into the minuteft veffels as being a preparation of iron, infinitely more fubtilized and attenuated, than in any of the preparations of that metal by art." Rutty on mineral Waters, p. 249. Virtues of Chalybeates.

There

There is also a small proportion of muriatic and earthy salt, mentioned above, but not in such proportion as to claim any share in the medicinal effects.

It is peculiarly adapted to promote appetite, and digestion, and to strengthen the tone of the stomach, impair'd by excess, or other causes It gradually strengthens the whole habit, and hence is excellent in that weakness, which remains after acute diseases, and for those who, without any apparent cause, lose their strength, fall away, and are commonly said to be going into a weakness. It is useful in the first stage, or beginning of consumptions, and may be used with advantage, even in the more advanced stages, if the matter spit up be good pus, and there be no considerable degree of fever.

It is of great service in nervous diseases, and in such as arise from weakness of the system, and reciprocally serve to increase it, as in the beginning of a dropsy, in the Fluor albus, or other seminal weaknesses, Diarrhæa, and Diabetes. It is good to prevent the gout in the stomach and bowels, may be useful in rheumatisms, and in some bodies to remove the causes of barrenness or imbecillity. In general, it will be serviceable

in

in a relaxed ftate of the folids, arifing from luxury, or excefs, inaction, or a fedentary life, or confequent on fome difeafe : it will correct a bad habit of body, and promote good fuppuration and granulation in ulcers ; and its frequent ufe will render a perfon lefs liable to be affected by cold, damp, or putrid air, epidemical or other caufes of difeafes. It will prove an efficacious medicine in all the cafes which were mention'd under the article of iron, p. 24, 25.

If the efcape of the fix'd air was prevented, we might alfo expect from it, in part, the virtues afcribed to that pervading principle. It may perhaps fometime prove of confequence enough, to have fome care taken to preferve its virtues entire, to be render'd (as it eafily might) more commodious and eafy of accefs, and to make it a matter of general joy, that a medicine of fuch public utility, is not in the hands of private men, who might circumfcribe its ufe, but a part of the public eftate and free to all comers.

U N F I T.

Thefe waters are unfit for old, infirm, perfons who have not heat enough to promote their action. The fame may be the cafe of fome *very weak* habits, and to fuch the exhibition of

the

the water fhould be very gradual, and prudently
regulated, it is not good for people, plethoric,
fat, difpos'd to inflammation or fpafmodic affec-
tion· and generally, where it heats much, it muft
either be omitted, or taken with proper precauti-
ons. To fome, a vomit, bleeding, or purging
may be neceffary, before entering on a courfe of
this water ; weak and delicate ftomachs may
require it diluted, or warm, or with the addition
of a little aromatic, or ftomach tincture, and in
fome, particularly the confumptive and gouty,
it will be proper to drink it with milk. Bark
infufed in it will in fome cafes be of fervice.
The body fhould in general be kept moderately
open during its ufe.

The METHOD OF USING THE WATER

The beft time for drinking this water is when
the ftomach is empty, in a morning, or an hour
or two before dinner. It is proper to begin
with half a pint, or a pint, and gradually to in-
creafe the dofe, fo as to take in fome cafes four
or five pints a day, or even to ufe it for common
drink at meals. The ufe of it fhould be continued for a pretty long time to reap the benefit
of it, and where the quantity drank has been
gradually increafed, as foon as the end propofed
is obtained, it fhou'd be gradually decreafed,
though not perhaps entirely left off. The fum-
mer

mer feafon is the beft for drinking it, altho' the chief reafon for this is, that it is the fitteft for exercife and bathing, which greatly promote the good effects of the water, efpecially in nervous cafes. this is alfo one motive for advifing its being drank at the fpring, rather than at home, Moderate exercife, regularity, temperance, a light, fimple, diet, not flatulent, ufing but little animal food, malt liquor, tea or coffee, and relaxation of the mind, alfo contribute much to affift its operation, as does, in obftructions, the warm bath.

§ 8. CASES.

AS a confirmation of what has been advanc'd of the good effects to be expected from the Liverpool Spà Water, I determined to collect fome cafes of perfons cured by its ufe, and to lay before the public fuch of them, as evinced moft clearly its efficacy. The three following, which I received from the patients, or their family, deferve particular attention, both by reafon of the confirm'd ftate of the difeafe, the imminent danger of the fick, and alfo as no other remedy being ufed at the fame time with the water, there is fufficient reafon to attribute to it alone, the furprizing change brought it about in the general ftate of health of each.

CASE

C A S E I.

Mifs Knowles, daughter of Mr. Knowles, in Caftle Ditch, had a fifter, who three years ago died of a confumption at the age of fixteen. A-bout a year afterwards, fhe herfelf, then twenty years old, was obferved to be in a decline. She complained of a bad cough, and great pain in her fide. She loft her flefh and her appetite en-tirely, and was defpaired of by the phyficians, whofe advice fhe followed long, but without be-nefit. Her father, tho' he believed there were no hopes remaining, yet recollecting that he had heard fome favourable accounts of our Liver-pool Spá Water, determin'd fhe fhould try that. He carried her up to it every morning, at firft with great difficulty. Within three days, howe-ver, fhe perceived good effects from its ufe and by a continuance of it, her appetite return'd, her digeftion was rendered good, fhe recovered her flefh, and ftrength, and is now perfectly well; yet ftill continues to drink the Spà Water occafion-ally, and attributing the prefervation of her life, and the recovery of her health folely to its ufe, has recommended it to numbers of people, who have alfo ufed it with confiderable benefit.

C A S E II.

Mifs Mofs of Middlewich, now Mrs. Eaton of Chefter, when about twenty, was thought to be in a comfumptive ftate. For two winters

fhe

she had been extremely emaciated, and had lived only on chocolate and oysters. She had so great a difficulty of breathing, and such violent pain in her side, as obliged her to walk bent double, and to seek relief from repeated bleeeding, even twice in a day. Her father (a judicious apothecary of Middlewich) almost despairing of her life, sent her to Liverpool on purpose to drink the Spà Water. She continued its use for some time with considerable benefit (taking no other medicine) and though her complaints were, both in their nature, duration, and violence, such as seemed to preclude every chance of recovery, yet she was soon restored to perfect health, and is now remarkably well and lusty.

C A S E   III.

Mr. Joseph Halfworth, aged about 50, brother in law to Mr. Yates, seedsman in Castle-street, for many years had laboured under a total want of appetite, digestion, and proper excretion, insomuch that frequently for a week together, he had no stool. Scarce a day passed but he vomited up a quantity of a black watry fluid, especially in an evening, and suffered grievously from a violent griping and twisting pain of the bowels, and at the pit of the stomach For the last ten years he had been much emaciated, and entirely incapable of working, or undergoing any fatigue. In this situation he came to Liverpool,

verpool, and in October 1772, began to drink
our Spá Water, induced by the many accounts
he heard of the good effects it had produced. In
a few days after he began to use it, his body became regularly open, his digestion good, his daily vomitings and colicky pains ceased entirely,
his appetite returned, he recovered in a short
time his flesh and strength, and has ever since
remained in a good state of health. He still continues to drink the water daily, and ascribes to it
alone the cure of his complaints; for, tho' he
had tried abundance of medicines, without effect
before he began to drink the water, yet he never
afterwards made use of any.

To these I might add a number of other
cases, less remarkable, in which it has been
found of signal service, but as I think the above
sufficient to prove its efficacy, and such as are
both perfectly indubitable and satisfactory, I
suppress many accounts I have received of persons who have been cured or relieved by the
Spá Water, in cases of loss of appetite, vomiting up the food, and general debility. Instances of this kind must have occurred to most of
my readers, within the circle of their acquain-
tance. Many such I have seen ; particularly a
friend of mine, who could never eat at breakfast
when he omitted drinking the water ; and a per-

H   son

fon troubled with indigeftion and frequent vomiting, who, tho' he is fo fituated as to have the
water brought to him, finds great benefit from
its ufe. But furely, enough has been faid, to
juftify a trial, and to prove, that 'tis no inconfiderable remedy in many cafes.

Thus have I endeavoured to explain clearly
and intelligibly, 1. the component parts, or che-
mical principles of the Liverpool Spá water, 2.
the medical virtues and good effects to be expected and derived from its ufe; and after pointing
out the cafes in which it may be of fervice, 3.
collected inftances in which it has.—I make no
doubt, but thefe might have been confiderably
augmented, and abundantly confirmed, by wait-
ing to obferve the fuccefs attending frefh trials of
it, and that thus, this work might have appeared
lefs incompleat and incorrect; but, as the feafon
for making ufe of it is now prefent, I chofe rather to fubmit thefe obfervations to the public,
crude and imperfect as they are, than to defer
exciting them to make trial of a remedy, in every
ones power, highly ufeful, and at once unex-
penfive and agreeable; happy if this attempt
may prove, in any degree, ferviceable to fociety.

Da veniam fcriptis, quorum non gloria nobis
   Caufa, fed utilitas, officiumque fuit.
                Ovid. 3. de Pont. Eleg. 9.

APPENDIX.

On the ACCIDENTAL USE of
LEAD.

Tanto pejus afficit, quo irrepit tectius.
BOERHAAVE, Elem. Chem. V. 2.

HAVING said so much, on what may not improperly be termed a *domestic medicine*, I shall take this occasion of cautioning the public against a *domestic poison*, the more to be apprehended, as its attacks are unperceived, and unsuspected, and its effects truly deplorable. Add to this, that there are few families, into which it does not, one way or other, find admission in a greater or less degree, and that, even in *very minute quantities*, it has been known to produce its bad effects on particular delicate constitutions. The pointing out so dangerous an enemy is of too much importance, not to render any apology unnecessary, for annexing. to this treatise, a few words on a subject no way connected with it.

LEAD

LEAD, by whatever means, or in whatever form it gains admittance into the human body, is found to produce dangerous or fatal effects. This seems to have been well known and perfectly underftood even by the antients; and Pliny, Ætius, Paulus Ægenita, and Vitruvius, have confidered Lead as highly poifonous. The Italians, French, &c. have long been wholly indebted to this metal, for thofe flow poifons, which were in former ages fo frequently adminifter'd, and which have render'd thofe nations fo defervedly infamous. By preparations of this metal they knew how to enfure death, even at a diftant period from their exhibition, or, by a continued, imperceptible, repetition of fmall dofes of them, to deftroy, without fufpicion, or the poffibility of detection. Shall we not then be aftonifh'd at being inform'd that we often are daily, of our own accord, fwallowing fmall dofes of this poifon, againft which we ought ever to be upon our guard?

We are indebted to the learned Dr. Baker for evincing, that the poifon of lead may, and frequently does, gain admittance into the human body, unobferved and unfufpected. The Dr has alfo been at great pains to caution the world againft it, by pointing out the

dangers

dangers attending it, and the various modes by which it may cafually gain admittance into the body ; fome of which are as follows.

1. In wines or cyder, with which lead is too frequently combined (particularly with the poorer, weak, acid, kinds) either intentionally and *fraudulently*, *cafually* and unnoticed, or *unfkilfully*. It has long been a practice with the makers or dealers in wine, when they find it poor, and difpofed to turn four, to add to it fome Ceruffe, Litharge, fugar of Lead, or other preparation of that metal , a practice, of which the noxious effects were fo notorious, that it was prohibited in France and Germany fince the year 1487, under pain of death. Yet, notwithftanding people are well apprized of the poifonous qualities communicated to the wine by this mixture, it is not uncommon to find the fmall, weak, white wines (as Lifbon, Rhenifh, Mofelle, French white) thus adulterated. It were well, if the Cyder-makers or venders were wholly free from this imputation. Certain it is, that cyder is often found adulterated with lead or its calces, which at once takes off any acidity it may have acquired, gives it a rich lufcious tafte, checks its fermenting, and improves its colour. Thefe effects have often given rife to the intentional and *fraudulent* mixture. But befides this, the fame

poifon

poison has been frequently added unknowingly
and *undesignedly*. If any lead vessels be used in
the preparation of cyder (as about the trough,
press, cistern, spouts &c.) the native acid of the
apple dissolves the metal, and forms with it su-
gar of lead, of which so small a portion, as six
or twelve grains, has been known to produce the
most terrible effects. In Devonshire particularly, lead was frequently employ'd in pre-
paring their cyder, and hence the metallic colic
is endemial, and the other effects of this poison
more frequent in that county, and the colic has
obtain'd amongst us the name of the Devonshire colic. Lead has also sometimes been combin'd with cyder, made-wines, &c. *unskillfully*,
by persons appriz'd of its correcting, and ignorant of its poisonous, quality. Thus hanging a
lead weight, or putting lead melted and pour'd
into water, in the cask, decanting the liquor into a leaden cistern; boiling it, before fermenta-
tion, in a copper, the upper part of which is of
lead; and even adding litharge; have been prac-
tised, and advised, as useful improvements, to
the great detriment of the families who have a-
dopted this custom, which, tho' recommended
in some cookery books, as a piece of good house-
wifery, for correcting any acid tendency in
wine, cyder, &c. has repeatedly proved fatal.
Several instances are produced by Dr. Baker of
metallic

metallic colics, palfies, and death, evidently occafion'd by this undefigned adulteration. Dr. Warren alfo mentions, that in the late Duke of Newcaftle's family, when at Hanover, in June 1752, thirty two perfons were feiz'd with the metallic colic, after having drank a fmall white wine, adulterated with lead. One of them died epileptic in lefs than a fortnight, the reft, after fuffering much and relapfing frequently, recover'd, except one, who remains paralytic. Even fhot remaining in bottles, and corroded by the liquor, may be of bad confequence. For certain it is, however the internal ufe of lead, as a medicine, may have been inculcated, in particular circumftances, by fome medical writers, it will generally be found to be, of a moft dangerous tendency.

The common wine meafures are made of bafe pewter, in which is a confiderable proportion of lead. Wine, cyder, or vinegar may prey upon thefe, and thus accidentally acquire a dangerous adulteration. The fame happens frequently from keeping thefe liquors in, or drinking them out of, common glazed earthen veffels.

The common black glaze is little elfe than an imperfect vitrification of lead; the common
yellow

yellow glaze, only a glafs of lead A fmall portion of lead is employ'd in glazing the earthen
ware, call'd Queens Ware, but is much more
difficultly foluble than in the two former. Stone
and flint ware only have a natural glaze, the
earth being vitrified by the addition of falt.
The lead is readily foluble in any acid liquor,
and fuch folutions become highly dangerous.
We all know, nothing is more common than to
keep pickles in black glaz'd earthen veffels ; yet
I believe it might be eafily proved, that vinegar
long kept therein, diffolves enough of the lead,
to render it not only an actual, but an active
poifon. This kind of glazed earthen ware
(and fometimes Pewter) is often ufed here
by the common people to bake fruit pies in,
and it is obferved, that the acid fruits take lefs
fugar to fweeten them, when baked in fuch.
The native vegetable acid, in this cafe, diffolves
a part of the lead, and is thereby corrected ;
but whoever is aware of the terrible effects, which
the fugar of lead, thus form'd, may produce
on the health, will always guard againft a practice, which to the generality appears both innocent, elegible and ufeful. Keeping milk, but-
termilk, fweetmeats, fyrups, or even moift fugar
in this kind of glazed earthen ware, is not void
of danger, as, by any thing difpofed to turn acid,
the glaze will be diffolved. On the fame principle

-ciple nothing can be more improper than fuch veffels, as are in general ufe amongft us, for fermenting fmall wines, as ginger wine, and treacle drink. Thefe large drink-pots, as they are called, are glazed on the infide with the common black glaze, and, as the fmall wines fermenting in them are, both from their weak nature, and the hot feafon in which they are chiefly ufed, particularly difpofed to become acid, this prevailing cuftom fhould be expofed as highly dangerous: and though it may not have been productive of confequences immediately alarming, yet it may have frequently given rife to weakneffes of the digeftive faculty, lofs of appetite, and complaints of the ftomach and bowels, which were never fufpected to arife from this caufe. Altho' fome conftitutions may, perhaps, not be injured by fuch repeated fmall dofes of this poifon, yet in delicate ones it may exert all its baneful influence: hence no one fhould expofe himfelf to it unneceffarily, and humanity requires our cautioning thofe ignorant of the danger, againft it. Nor are the common glazed platters proper for baking or falting meat, as the lead is foluble in greafy fubftances, and may be corroded by the falt. Glafs, ftone, and flint ware, being void of danger, fhould be fubftituted inftead of glazed veffels for the above purpofes.

I

It

It is almoſt a conſtant practice to prepare our food, in copper veſſels *tinned*; the metal with which they are lined, conſiſts of above ⅐ part of lead, which diſſolves not only in acids, but even in oil, butter or greaſe, particularly if ſuffered to ſtand in them.

I have been aſſured by Profeſſor Gaubius, in Holland, that the people there, have ſometimes endeavoured to encreaſe the weight of their butter, by adding to it a calx of lead; but I hope, and believe, no ſuch diabolical practice prevails in England.

New rum is found to be alſo accidentally impregnated with lead, and to produce the metallic colic, or dry belly-ach, as it is call'd in the Weſt Indies, where it is frequent from this cauſe; not, as was ſuſpected, from the great uſe of acids. for acids are even found to be the beſt defence againſt the bad effects of ſuch ſolutions of lead. But when it is known, that " the juice of the ſugar cane, when expreſſed, flows into a veſſel lined with lead; that leaden gutters, or pipes, are uſed to convey it to the boiling houſe, and the ſkimmings and molaſſes from thence to the ſtill-houſe, that the ſugar coppers are rimmed with lead; the ſtill is copper, tinn'd; and the ſtill-head and worm are of tin or common pewter, and the latter (till of late years) of lead,"

it

ir will not be wonder'd at, if new rum fhould be found to contain a portion of this metal. By keeping the rum (as alfo wine and cyder) this is decompofed and precipitates, fo that thefe liquors grow lefs dangerous on that fcore by age.

Lead, in general, is not diffolv'd by water, but fometimes, by long ftanding and attrition, is mix'd with, and fufpended in it, in a very fine powder, by no means innocent, tho' not near fo dangerous as when 'tis diffolv'd by an acid. It is not however quite clear, that certain waters may not be impregnated with acid, or faline, principles, which may render them capable of diffolving lead, and thus becoming an active poifon. Dr Wall gives an inftance of a gentleman of Worcefter, who had twenty children, of whom eight died young. The reft during their infancy, and until they quitted the houfe they liv'd in, were all remarkably unhealthy, and fubject to diforders of the ftomach and bowels. The father was many years paralytic, the mother, fubject to colics and bilious obftructions (which were reliev'd by Bath waters, but return'd when fhe came back to her own houfe) died of the jaundice. When the houfe was fold, and the lead pump came to be repair'd, the cylinder was much worn, and the ciftern was fo corroded as not to be thicker than paper, and was full of holes,

though

though the pump had been feveral times repair'd, even but 3 or 4 years before, when it was nearly in the fame ftate. The water of that place is very hard, and hence probably corroded readily the lead, and becoming ftrongly impregnated with that metal, was the unfufpected caufe of the ill health of this family, for many years.

As this circumftance may caufe a diftruft of the water with which many families are fupplied, I fhall here add an eafy method, by which the mixture of lead with other fubftances may, at any time, readily be difcovered. Take pot afh, and fulphur, equal parts, and boil them together in water for half an hour : add, very gradually, a little of this liquor to the water you would examine, and a cloudinefs will appear ; if lead is contain'd, the colour, and precipitated powder, will be dark grey ; if no lead be contain'd, they will be white and milky ; and the darkifh fhade will be greater or lefs, in proportion to the greater or lefs quantity of lead contain'd, as may be feen by adding a little fugar of lead, to water intended for examination and comparifon.

A caution feems to be neceffary againft feeding children with pewter fpoons, which are made of bafe metal, contain much lead, and

are

are too often fuffer'd to ftand in the milk, &c.
which the child takes: as alfo againft giving them
toys daub'd with paint to amufe them, in which
lead has a great fhare ; young children generally
putting into their mouths whatever they have
in their hands. Hence, not improbably, may
arife many of thofe complaints in the ftomach
and bowels which are frequent in infants, who will
be much eafier affected, than others, by the noxious metal. Nor muft we lofe fight of this, that,
as the action of this poifon is on the nervous fyftem, its effects will be very different in different
conftitutions, and the fame dofe will frequently
caufe no fenfible bad effect on fome, which may
fuffice to produce the moft deplorable evils, and
even incurable complaints in others. And
hence it is, that thefe confequences of an accidental ufe of lead are not fo general, as we might
otherwife expect them to be --But as a proof that
thefe combinations of lead are not fuppofition
only, real lead can be obtain'd from them.

Lead even externally applied has proved hurtful, altho' it is the bafis of an external remedy
againft inflammation, &c, which is of infinite
ufe when prudently adminifter'd, acts on the
nervous fyftem, and takes off inflammation, ob-
tunding the fenfibility. A piece of fheet lead
worn upon an iffue, a plaifter of which lead is

the

the principal ingredient, a poultice, or an in-
jection of a folution of lead, have, in certain irritable habits, produced effects, fimilar to thofe
confequent on the internal ufe of it. Even duft-
ing the excoriated parts of children with white
lead, has been known to caufe convulfions.

The complaints confequent on the ufe of lead,
are frequent amongft thofe whofe bufinefs expofes them to the action of this metal, as plumbers,
potters, painters, glafs-grinders, &c. Even prin-
ters by ufing their types, when too much heated in
drying, have been known to feel the bad effects
of the effluvia of lead. For " lead whether diffolved by fire or corroded by an acid, emits
poifonous effluvia " In the cutting of glafs a
leaden wheel is ufed, and the vapor arifing from
thence is known to be highly hurtful to the
workmen employ'd at it, who are fubject to the
metallic colic, and frequently become paralytic.
By a greater degree of heat, lead emits more
and more dangerous effluvia, which act often
with equal, if not greater violence, than its preparations taken internally. Even the heat of the
atmofphere alone caufes it to emit a baneful vapor. Inftances are not wanting where living in
a room which has been newly painted (efpecially
white) has caufed thefe complaints, and birds,
&c. fhut up in it, have died. The vapor from

oil

oil-cafe (which has fugar of lead in its compofition) may produce inconveniences to delicate
habits, particularly to fuch as wear focks of it.

The *effects* confequent upon this accidental
ufe of lead, are, obftinate conftipation, with
violent colicky pains (the Colica Pictonum, De-
vonfhire, or more properly, *metallic colic*) and
confequent paralytic affections, refolution and
lofs of colour of the mufcles, pains, tremors,
fpafms, fuppreffion of urine, afthma, fuffocati-
on; vertigo, epilepfy, apoplexy, idiotifm;
pulmonary confumption, flow fever and death.

Thofe whofe employment expofes them to the
action of poifonous metallic effluvia, as thofe
who work in lead mines, copper works, &c.
find the beft preventative to be greafy fubftances, as fat broth or oil taken every morning, and thus they are in fome degree defended
againft its baneful influence.

For the *cure* of the metallic colic, recourfe is
had to the Cremor Tartari, Caftor Oil, fometimes to the quick, active, purgatives, emetics
opiates and glyfters. The Bath waters are found
very ferviceable in palfies confequent on this metallic colic. Very excellent effects are related by
Grafhuis, and after him, by our ingenious

coun-

countryman Dr. Percival of Manchefter, from roch alum, fifteen grains, given every four or five hours, in the metallic colic, which the latter fays has, in fifteen cafes, fucceeded with him, relieving the pain, and the fecond or third dofe proving aperient.---But nothing gives fo immediate temporary relief, as the warm bath; yet it fhould be long continued, and occafionally repeated, to prove of permanent advantage. Its ufe calms, removes fpafms, and difpofes the body to be fooner acted upon, by the medicines employ'd to get the better of the conftipation.

A woman of this town, from the ufe of paint was afflicted grievoufly with the metallic colic, and had, for feveral days, tried a variety of means to procure relief, under the direction of a fkilful and experienced phyfician, but with little fuccefs. Defpairing almoft of his patient's recovery, he mention'd the cafe to me, and we jointly determined to try the warm bath. She fat in it near an hour, and experienced an almoft immediate ceffation of pain; and though this was not durable, a repetition of the warm bath, with proper aperient medicines, foon effected a cure. It is remarkable, that in the fame houfe, from the like cuftom (painting) there were two women fubject to epileptic complaints.

As

As the practice of painting the face, is by no means prevalent here, I thought it unneceffary to add any caution on this head. But it may not be amifs to remark, that in France, where this cuftom is general, they themfelves are fenfible of the mifchiefs occafion'd by it, particularly by the cheaper and more ordinary kinds of *rouge*, which confift chiefly of lead. But the greateft danger to be apprehended is from the *white*, which they rub into the fkin, to hide the natural dimnefs of their complexions.

Nor are the ill effects of this metal confin'd to man alone. the brute creation are equally liable to be affected by it, from accidental caufes, as feeding from leaden veffels, or drinking water impregnated with lead. The cattle which feed, or drink, in the neighbourhoood of furnaces for fmelting lead, and the cats of plumbers, and others who work in lead, are remarkably fubject to colics, and to a gradual decay.

Thus have I curforly enumerated, the various means by which the poifon of lead may, and does infinuate itfelf into the body, and endeavour'd to caution the public againft a dangerous and unfufpected enemy; and I would humbly hope, that, however foreign from my fubject this may appear, the attempt will, in fome degree, prove both agreeable and ferviceable to my readers

F I N I S.

CPSIA information can be obtained at www.ICGtesting.com
Printed in the USA
LVOW052031210113

316601LV00012B/756/P

9 781170 013052